Healing The Woman Within

Blending Functional Medicine And Intuitive Healing

By Dr. Alison DiBarto Goggin

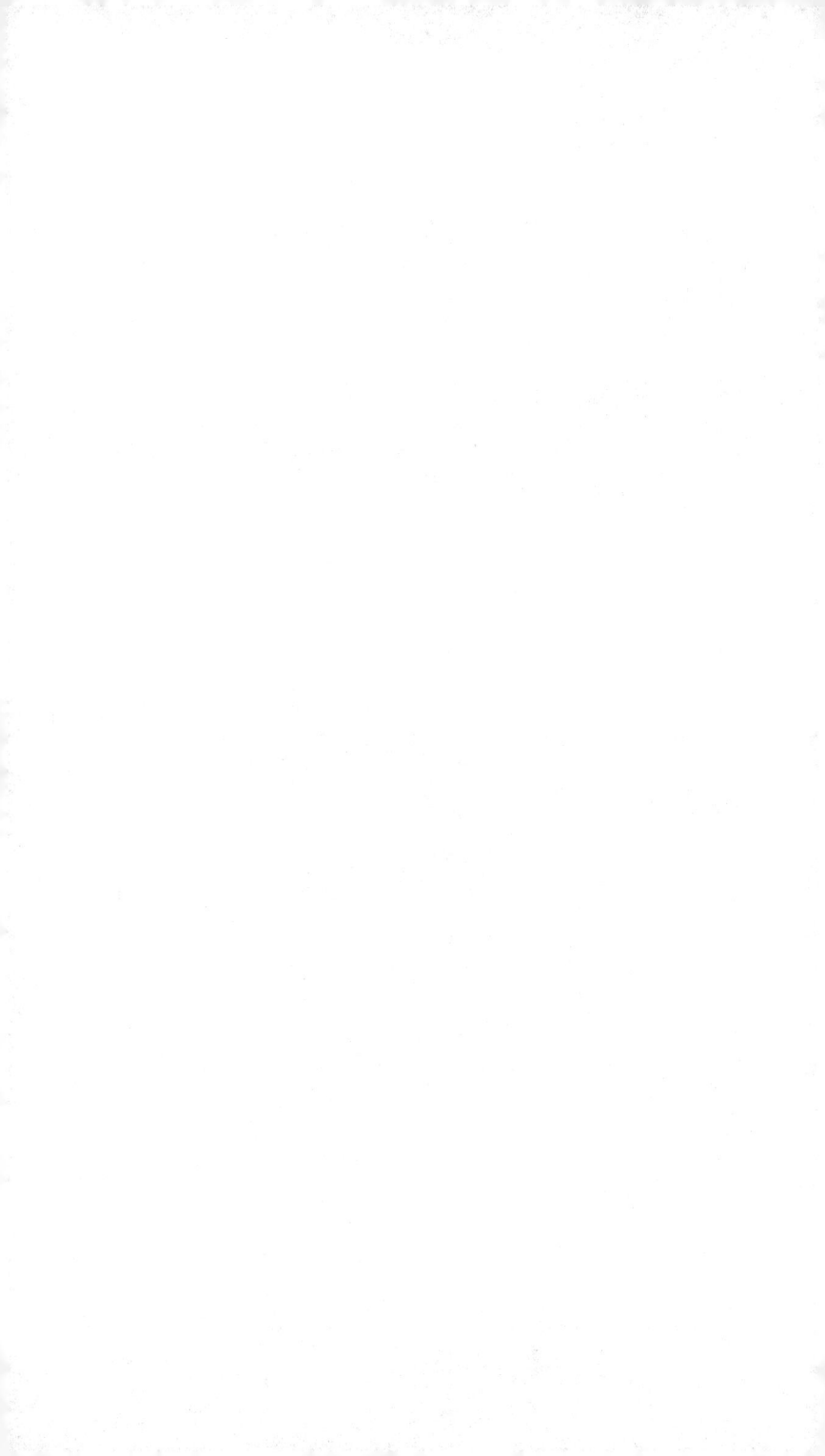

Copyright © 2018 Dr. Alison DiBarto Goggin
All rights reserved.
ISBN: 9781791685812

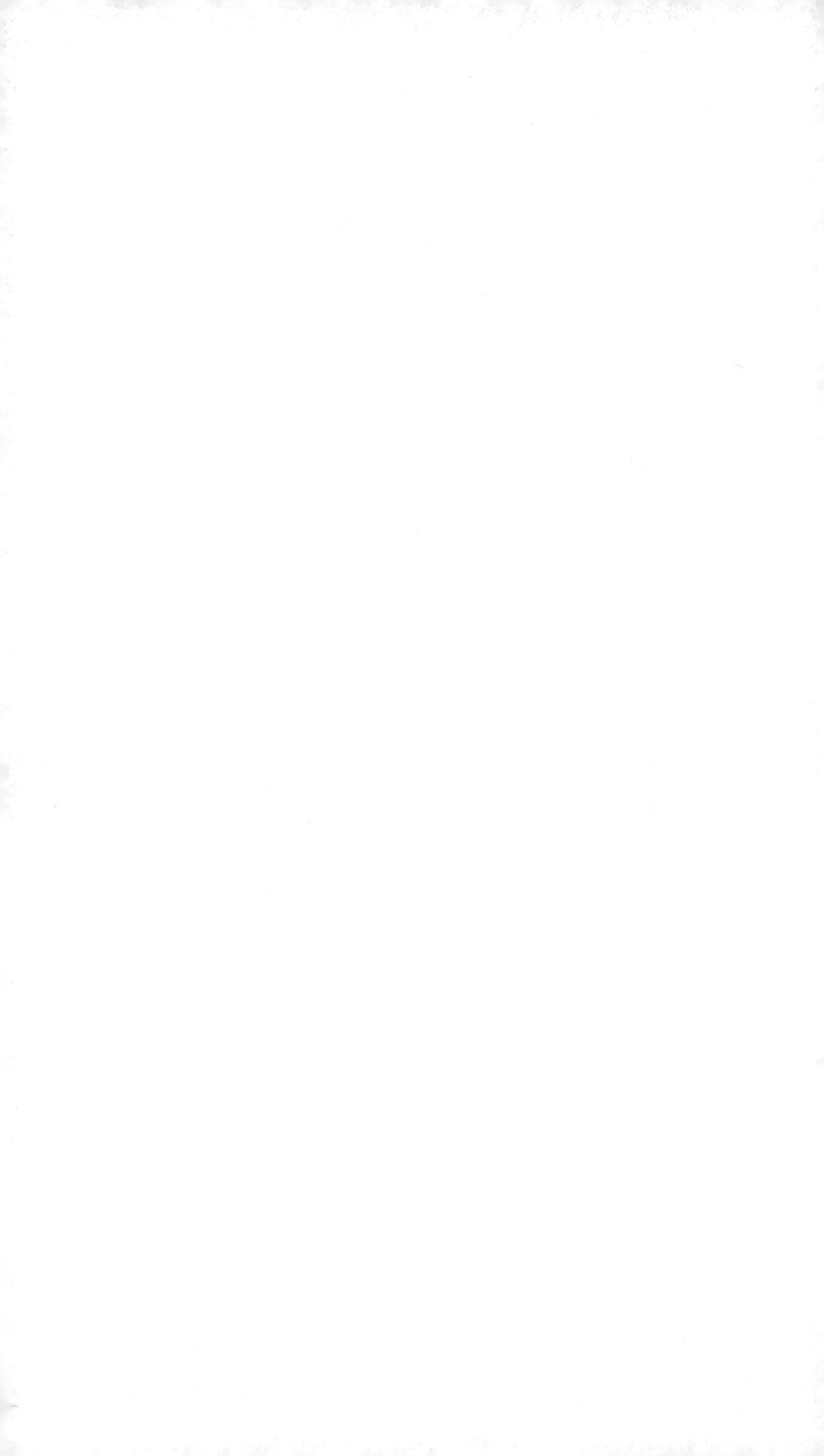

Dedicated to my sister family
Who are looking for answers
To find hope, peace, and healing

Healing The Woman Within
Introduction 9
Chapter 1: Introducing The Problem   15
Chapter 2: Stop Guessing   25
Chapter 3: Putting The Pieces Together 32
Chapter 4: The Real You   40
Chapter 5: Everyone Else   47
Chapter 6: Your Spirit   68
Chapter 7: Your Intuition   81
Chapter 8: The Unending Journey   89
About The Author   92

Introduction

This is not a how-to book, a meal plan, or your next best thing to lose weight quick. This book is about finding the truth about your health, what is blocking you from healing, and thinking about your body from a different perspective.

There are two days in my life that terrified me and forced me to question everything I knew about my body and traditional medicine. These experiences have helped me become a lighthouse leader and healer. I want my stories and strategies to stand as a lighthouse, a beacon of hope for when you are lost, confused, sad, and alone. Follow the light because you know that path has already been traveled by many before you. As a culture we share stories, some are driven to save you from suffering in the hopes you will heed their lessons.

Others share stories because they know that everyone suffers, life's struggles and pain are shared by everyone, but through our stories and healing we can show others how to overcome more quickly, show the paths that can be walked as you choose how you want to move forward in your life.

My journey really started when I was 15 and was struggling with chronic and severe leg pain in both of my legs. I quit swimming because my shoulder pain and joined track. I quickly developed stress fractures in both of my legs that healed but the pain never stopped. We had tried everything on the traditional medicine list and the next step was an electromyography. This test was described to me as "we are going to put needles in your leg and make you walk on a treadmill".

I almost vomited in the car on the long drive to the office and about fell over with joy when the doctor told me we could skip it. That story didn't improve much from there but I was allowed to live without that test but the pain was relentless and I was prescribed anti-depressants and sleeping pills. I spent the next few years struggling with suicidal depression, anxiety, and in and out of psychiatrists offices.

I vividly remember sitting at the rheumatologists office, looking out the window as he talked on and on about nothing, and I thought about how I could throw myself out the window and die. Sleeping pills, antidepressants, and birth control should never have been options for me, and when those doctors knew what they were doing to me I should have been tapered off.

I didn't know anything about natural health, supplements, or energy medicine and my parents certainly didn't. We all did the best we could for my body at that time and I see this part of my story the set up for how I could help others who struggle with anxiety, depression, insomnia, and stress see the light of the other side.

The proof in my ability to heal was revealed when I was 26. During an annual check up I was forced to sign a waiver stating that I had cancer, I refused to follow the recommended protocol, and I was going to die. The nurse wrote and circled "CANCER" and "DEATH" on the waiver in bright red pen. A few months before that day I was diagnosed with cervical dysplasia and had not followed up after my initial treatment. Instead, I chose to use an herbal treatment alongside of nutrition, energy healing, and chiropractic.

I had no idea if my protocol would work, but I trusted in myself, my body, and my training. At my cancer/death appointment I was told I would get a call with my results in a week, the next treatments were outlined for me because I was told I certainly had cancer that progressed and I needed more intense treatment. After two weeks without a call, I called the office expecting the worst. I was sternly told by the nursing staff that they don't call patients who have normal results and she hung up. I have always had a normal pap since that day!

As I continued my education through chiropractic college, functional medicine courses, nutrition, and applied kinesiology I learned how the body truly works at to start asking questions rather than providing protocols. I love chiropractic, I still adjust my family and see my own chiropractor, but I didn't agree with the philosophy that an adjustment will fix all sources of illness all of the time. I wanted to be the doctor who had the private office for my patient's to come in, tell me about their pain in a safe and honored space.

When I was at a kinesiology seminar I told my friend about my unrelenting shoulder pain that had returned from my swimming days. He laughed when I told him all my serious diagnoses that I was given and went to work with me. He helped me understand that my gallbladder was referring pain to my shoulder because I wasn't digesting fats very well and that my liver was congested with hormones.

I started my plan with enzymes and support and in a few days I was pain free. To this day I know when my shoulder acts up I need to watch the types of fat I am eating and make sure I take my enzymes. This experience brought me fully into functional medicine as I learned more about how our organs, spine, hormones, and food are all related and how we can find the root cause first.

I hope that this book helps you understand the layers of how your body works, how your symptoms correlate to each other, that you can test and stop guessing why you are feeling ill, and the experiences, environments, and your intuition all play a major role in your healing.

Chapter 1: Introducing The Problem

In this book we will start with the physical aspects of health and healing and lead into the emotional and spiritual aspects. In traditional medicine we focus only on the body and how to mask symptoms, with functional medicine we focus on finding and addressing the root cause, and in whole body healing we focus on the emotions and trauma that have been stored and are harming our body.

Your physical pain is real though many friends and physicians have told you it isn't. Something has changed in your body even if your test results are 'normal'. If your body is giving you a message that something is wrong, you are experiencing symptoms that aren't going away, then there is a true physiological process going on.

Most of my patients come to me asking
"What is wrong with me"
"Why isn't anything working"
"What if I never feel good again"
"Why doesn't my doctor have answers"

We are told to ignore our deepest concerns because it seems too crazy or wild. We suppress our body's functions with medicines to conceal what is actually going on. On the other extreme some will just assume they are irrational, stressed, and label themselves as a hypochondriac. They never seek help and look only to emotional support to cure their symptoms and most of this these coping methods include alcohol, drugs, checking-out with television or their phones.

The underlying problem for women who are chronically ill, tired, and down is that we are disconnected from our bodies because we are disconnected from our soul. We are all innately built with intuition, a gut feeling, a fleeting thought or dream but we have been conditioned to ignore our soul and some have even been taught that trusting yourself is evil. Living without intuition has us consumed with our culture, judgemental and angry with everyone around us, shut off from our bodies and natural cycles.

Women are suffering with unexplainable and untreatable anxiety, depression, no interest in sex or connection, and are blindly moving through life in a constant state of overwhelm and stress. We live with no focus, no meaning, and the light in our souls grows dimmer.

Fear of following our intuition has cost us dearly. We live in a 'what if' state always afraid of making a mistake, looking foolish, or losing everything we cherish. Freedom is unsafe, intuition is a false feeling, and we hold on tighter to the material life we have created. We are so consumed with the culture of stress it is the only way we find connection. Meeting up with friends becomes a contest over who is struggling more, who is taking more medication, and who has the most drama in their relationships.

We only find connection in chaos.

We have forgotten how to share our dreams, ideas, our creativity. Somewhere in our lives we were shut down and we were never taught how to recover, regain balance, and find strength.

We are cut off from the woman within.

Asking the question "who are you" is traumatizing, riddled with stories of who we are supposed to be, wanted to be, conditioned to be by our family, religion, and culture. We aren't sure how to answer that question when you take away the relationship labels of wife, mother, daughter, teacher, lawyer, etc.

If you were to shed the stories of who you think you are supposed to be, release the labels of relationships and jobs, who are you?

Who would you be if you were standing in your own power, your true self, and your soul was shining through?

Our feminine powers of protecting, providing, creating, birthing, caring, and loving deeply have been suppressed to keep us safe from expanding too far into the unknown. It's not safe to travel, leave your job, leave your abusive relationship, start a business, go to school, ask for help. We ignore the calling of our soul to fly free, experiment, create, and love.

What does any of this have to do with healing and functional medicine?

Being cut off from the woman within has cut us off from our intuition, our body, and our health. Women are racing from doctor to doctor, prescriptions to surgery, therapist to the gym, looking for answers to cure their anxiety and pain but rarely find a solution.

Intuition as I use the term here is the instinctive voice within yourself. You may call it your gut feeling or your heart talking. You may feel a pull when you know something is off, that person next to you isn't safe, or you feel like you will be sick if you have to be around that group of people.

It may look like you applying for a job or to a school on a 'whim', or picking out this book, or starting up a conversation with someone across the room at a coffee shop. You feel a pull or sensation that tells you what you should do next.

For years I chased the labels of adrenal fatigue, leaky gut, hormone imbalances, anxiety, and depression. I was experiencing severe fatigue, brain fog, muscle weakness, and difficulty balancing hormones. I consulted many different types of physicians and healers and I was told that I had adrenal fatigue and I needed more energy work, acupuncture, herbs, foods, you name it to relax and support my adrenals.

I was muscle tested for low iron, sometimes thyroid, sometimes leaky gut. I was told I was just sabotaging myself because I would start a new exercise program and two weeks later I would be weak and sick. I was even told that I intuitively knew what was going on and I just needed to meditate. But I knew there was something deeper going on and I hadn't looked far enough.

When I had my labs done I found out that I had iron overload and my iron saturation was also extremely high. I asked five functional medicine physicians what they thought of my blood work and they all gave me five completely different answers. One even told me nothing was wrong!

I knew in my heart but also from my training to look for a gene that is related to iron overload so I went back to the lab trusting my instincts. I found out a few days later that I did have one of the genes that was linked to my high iron! I was so relieved and the big picture of my symptoms became clear.

I was experiencing weakness right before my period because my iron was so high, plus I was taking iron supplements because I muscle tested as needing them. This caused my muscles and joints to weaken, my fatigue escalated, and pain in my liver. Then when I had my period and released the excess iron I felt better. I always thought it was incredibly strange but it wasn't until I had my blood work done that I finally had the right answers. I still have to focus on my foods, eating clean and in the right time, supporting my body with nutrition and essential oils, but finding this major piece of the puzzle has changed everything. Plus, I can stop blaming myself for 'sabotaging' and feeling down on myself when I know that there is a true cause.

Chasing the wrong diagnosis and treatment is what many people experience before they find the right answer. Doctor's are not always right and they definitely aren't always right on the first try.

We have to peel back the layers of someone's health and work one step at a time. Of course you have to address what seems most obvious and work through the layers of the body, but you can also have tests done and not blame your emotional state as the sole cause of all of your symptoms. Trust yourself!

My passion is listening to women and finding the core of their pain, both physical and emotional. Many times I am the only person who believes that their anxiety is not in their head but there is a true physical cause as well. Women are largely ignored in the medical community, a blanket prescription of birth control and antidepressants is the mainstream way of managing symptoms, and by the way eat less food please. Women are dying after giving birth in alarming rates in the United States because their cries for help are ignored and labeled as over dramatic, weakness, and attention seeking.

Women have shut down their interaction with their bodies and their intuition because everyone else knows more than and better than they ever will. Your doctor hates that you research before you come in the office, your husband is convinced you need to just be consistent, and your friends think you're lazy. While deep down you know none of it is true.

When you are cut off from your body and intuition, you suppress your natural instincts and urges. This often manifests in the relationship with food. Women starve themselves, they tell me that they just aren't hungry. Other women binge and overeat, suppressing the signal to stop eating or find healing emotional coping methods.

After a short amount of time your cells will change and become suppressed as well. Your brain has a group of neurons (paraventricular nucleus) that monitors the blood and adjusts hormones and signals accordingly. When you suppress the signals for hunger, movement, connection, this group of neurons learns that it is on it's own and starts to run your body without your input, usually causing adrenal fatigue and insulin resistance. Your cells will build calcium shells and stop accepting hormone instructions and nutrition.

By fearing rejection and cutting ourselves off from our source we subconsciously reject our body and bring illness, pain, and emotional disruption.

While I do believe that many illnesses are based in harmful emotional patterns, I do not believe that all diseases can be caused and cured by emotional and psychological healing. We do not have to blame someone for their illness because of their emotions.

In my opinion, illness can be considered a chicken-or-the-egg situation where we have environmental factors that can cause disease and our emotions exacerbate them through inflammation and hormone interaction and vice versa. I still focus on treating both the physical and emotional body because we cannot separate the two.

Take the time to journal on these questions as you think about your health, your symptoms, how you are feeling right now and how you would like to feel in the future.

- How do you feel right now in your body? How do your muscles, joints, and spine feel? What is your energy level? Are you comfortable sitting here or tense?
- How would you love to feel in your body? Not just weight, but as you move through your day, cook food, and show up at work.
- What do you think is holding you back from achieving this vision for yourself?
- How do you recognize your intuition? Do you feel a pull in your heart, do you have a sense of knowing, do thoughts just come through or do you hear that small voice share words?
- How do you respond to your intuition? Do you always follow the guidance or do you ignore the feelings because logically and consciously the ideas don't make sense?
- What do you think would happen if you always followed your intuition? Would life

be more difficult and confusing, would scary truths arise, or would life be easier to navigate when you trust yourself?
- Sit quietly and reflect on what can you do this week to connect to your intuition.
- Now that you are connected to your body and self, ask again, what do you think is holding you back from achieving this vision for yourself?

Chapter 2: Stop Guessing

She walks in my office and drops down two grocery bags onto my adjusting table. "Here is everything I'm taking, can you muscle test me on each one and tell me how much I need to take?" I hate these days at my office. People are wasting hundreds of dollars because of what they read is amazing on the latest blog or running through the nutrition stores talking to employees that have never been trained and aren't asking them the right questions.

As I muscle tested this person through every bottle I asked her why she purchased each one and what is was for. She had no answers she just 'heard it was good'. In the end she left with instructions to take 3 of those bottles on a daily basis and toss the rest because they were chemically based, non-food pills that her body wouldn't absorb and we found out a few of her adrenal support herbs were actually causing more harm after her cortisol tests came back.

You might be the person who is educated, empowered, savvy, and loves to research, keep it up. You need to know that every symptom you have cannot be healed with an herb or nutrient that some expert has on their blog and in their store.

You buy the latest health book and by the time you are done with all the symptoms quizzes you are convinced you have every disease, gene mutation, and hormone dysfunction and will probably die tomorrow.

You can buy every supplement you can hoping that this one will be the answer to your pain, insomnia, suffering, but we have all been down this path. Even my pantry is filled with supplement bottles! Your friends are selling the latest shake, drink, powder, and pill with promises of reclaiming your youthful energy. Yet, each one only helps for a short amount of time or doesn't make any difference at all. Why do your friends look so good and you feel so sick still? You start wondering why you are even bothered to keep trying to find the support you desperately need.

The first key here is to stop.

Stop going to the nutrition store and asking your friends what they use. Stop buying supplements, powders, and pills. Nothing can address your issues until you know exactly what they are, until then, you are just guessing.

And most importantly stop buying supplements online unless they are directly from the retailer. Anyone can buy a supplement bottle and refill it with anything, put a safety seal on it and sell you something that could harm you. Many of my friends were buying their probiotics online, until they called the retailer to ask why they weren't shipped cold with a pack. The company said they didn't sell online and to never buy those again, who knows what was in those bottles!

Though I strongly believe in and practice muscle testing, aka applied kinesiology, we have to stop relying on that as our only method of testing. Don't be the person in the aisle swaying back and forth thinking that is your body giving you an answer. When I hear someone tell me they practice that type of 'muscle testing' I have to tell them that the swaying is happening because their pelvis needs to be adjusted and they have a category I or II dysfunction. I love you and there are better options.

How do you test your body to know exactly what is going on with every system?

In functional medicine, we say "Don't Guess, Test", which means starting with a basic blood test to evaluate the body as a whole. From there we can order more tests as we find issues or even unique testing like stool, saliva, urine, and hair.

The most common phrase I hear from every patients is "my doctor says my blood work is normal but I still feel sick, how can that be?". The reason that your blood work appears to be healthy is because the traditional lab ranges are very large and set by the lab for that local geographic region. A bell curve is applied to the ranges that the lab collects throughout the year so anything in the middle is considered 'normal' and anything outside of that is considered 'abnormal'. This means only 5% of a range is considered outside of normal limits.

To you, this means that your blood tests are coming back normal because you are just like 95% of your population, who are also not one hundred percent healthy.

Functional medicine uses much smaller ranges that we consider to be truly a healthy range. Results that are between the functional abnormal and medical normal are considered to be a physiological trend towards disease, and values outside of the medical ranges of normal are true pathology.
This allows us to see where your body is beginning to struggle before medical intervention such as prescriptions or surgery are needed.

When Michelle started a program with my office she had all the classic hypothyroid issues. Her hair was falling out, she couldn't lose weight, her fatigue was so significant that she rarely made it to work on time.

She was convinced that she had a thyroid issue but her TSH level was 'normal' and nothing else was tested or recommended except for the classic "lose weight, eat less, workout". I went ahead and ordered her a full thyroid panel (TSH, all the T4's and T3's) plus the autoimmune antibodies.

I'm sure you can guess that while her TSH was normal by the lab standards, by functional standards she was 3 points above our normal ranges. She also had positive antibodies to her thyroid and her low iron was part of her hair falling out. After her program she has been able to stop the hair loss, she released 15 pounds, and her thyroid labs are within a completely normal range!

The next caveat to your blood work is that many physicians refuse to order whole panels for the thyroid and liver, leaving you without vital information. Many times this is because they are restricted by their place of work or insurance coverage and they are doing their best within their restricted environments.

When I review my patient's 'normal' bloodwork I often find results that are within medical ranges but outside of our functional ranges and we are able to start understanding which underlying systems are struggling.

I personally know how frustrating this whole process is when you are looking for answers. Remember my story of when I finally had my own blood panel tested. Somehow I had let 10 years go by without any blood work! When I got my results back I had a the issues with my iron and I bet you can guess what answers I received when I asked 5 doctors what it meant. I got 5 completely different answers. I had to go back for more testing to see what was actually happening. The moral of this story is that you should keep testing, don't accept 'normal' as an answer when you know there is something truly going on with your body.

There have been amazing advances in the science of testing the body and it's systems. When I first learned about leaky gut it was considered fad science, there was no way to test for it so how can we prove it? Now, we have the marker Zonulin that we can test to determine the health of the gut barrier. We have incredible research on autoimmune conditions and the organs that are at risk. Women commonly and unknowingly struggle with ovarian destruction with autoimmune complications.

If your blood work comes back normal you should know about alternative testing options:
- Food sensitivity testing through blood
- Saliva testing for hormone patterns
- Saliva testing to track your cortisol through the day
- Genetic testing
- Nutritional status testing
- Parasite, yeast, fungal testing
- Specific toxin testing
- Autoimmune testing for every system in the body

A starting option for you today is to take a functional medicine systems quiz. Click this link to take the systems survey quiz online at www.standardprocess.com/Systems-Survey and email me your results at YourOilDoc@gmail.com.

Chapter 3: Putting The Pieces Together

My job as a functional medicine physician is to play detective as well as an annoying but curious toddler. I ask "why" over and over until we find the true root cause behind someone's myriad of symptoms.

I had a friend come to me who was having a lot of different issues, but her main concern was that she was gaining weight. As I talked to her, we started to go through some symptoms that she was having and the list was forever long. She was having pain on her right side right where her ribs were, she was struggling with varicose veins, acne, psoriasis, diverticulitis, which is a gut issue, hormone imbalances and hemorrhoids.

All these things together, it looks complicated, it feels complicated. When she went to what I call specialized medicine, which is traditional medicine, her GI specialist took out her gallbladder, her gynecologist recommended birth control, her primary care recommended sleeping pills.

Chiropractic, physical therapy, and massage didn't help with her pain and she was stuck living with all of this. She accepted that there was really nothing she could do and she was just getting old. Varicose veins are part of life. Acne, part of life. Psoriasis, she was given a cream.

Her blood work looked great, and they told her just to eat clean, and she was given a total hysterectomy when she was 26 and put on birth control and hormones. Then of course with the weight gain she was just told, well, exercise more. None of these are options that helped her feel better. None of these got rid of the pain or the hormone imbalance.

With my training and detective work, I get to look at all of these symptoms and put it together. From a functional perspective, all of these symptoms looked like liver to me. The pain on the right side, that's where her liver was, and we have to think about the organs when someone isn't responding to chiropractic or physical therapy. And what happens with hormone imbalance, specifically, is that the hormones build up and build up in the liver. You know of estrogen dominance, which causes heavy periods, lots of bleeding, clotting, major PMS symptoms, you're on the couch for days because you can't stop bleeding, and then you're told well, let's just get rid of your uterus. Or let's do an ablation, or here's some birth control and some antidepressants.

These issues back up the liver, and when the liver backs up, it swells the veins. So when you have something like varicose veins and hemorrhoids, we know that's probably a liver issue.

Then the diverticulitis because as the hormones go through the liver into the gallbladder, it irritates the gallbladder, and then it irritates the digestive tract as your body's trying to get rid of all these excess hormones, and it just can't function. And how can you lose weight when your liver isn't functioning, your hormones are overwhelmed, nothing is being processed. And of course, psoriasis, to me, always originates from the liver.

I asked her to go to our local nutrition store and pick up three supplements. Those are specific to her, so I don't want to say exactly what they are because all of my protocols are specific to each specific patient. Two weeks after she started her protocol, she sent me a text and said she's been taking the cleanse every day, and the enzymes, and she's noticed a 110% difference. "I can't thank you enough for helping me."

It really irritates her that she was put on birth control when that wasn't even the problem. So many women have this story of my doctor wrote me off, they say oh, your bleeding to death, that's just normal, you'll have to live with it, when it's not normal. It might be common, those experiences are very, very common, but it is not normal.

Another common complaint that I hear is "why is nothing working for me"? I worked with a friend who had asthma. She was on every asthma medication, she was using every essential oil, she was taking all of the right supplements. I worked with a nurse who felt like she was having a heart attack, and it happened about three times a month, and her EKGs were normal, her blood work was normal, her X-rays, everything that she tested was normal. My husband suffered with shoulder pain, and chiropractic didn't help, massage, he had MRIs, which came back looking great, ultrasounds, ultrasounds looked great. So why is nothing working for them?

Specialized medicine can only provide their tools which are surgery and prescriptions. For asthma, she was given the drugs. For the heart attack please go to the emergency room. With shoulder pain, like I said, therapy, injections, chiropractic, are amazing. We need all of these things, and drugs can be so supportive when they're necessary, and supporting the right symptom. Therapy and injections can be so amazing, but if it's not addressing the root cause, then you're not going to get better.

For all of these people, they ended up having the same issue, which was acid reflux. For asthma, the acid reflux was coming up when she was sleeping, and then going into her lungs and causing irritation, so she would wake up and hack, and have difficulty breathing, which is why the drugs and the oils weren't working. My friend who was having the heart attack, she was drinking coffee and eating some really unhealthy foods because she was at work, and that's all she could get her hands on which was causing reflux, but because of the pain it felt enough to call it a heart attack, especially on that left side. With my husband's shoulder pain he was experiencing referral pain from acid reflux because the stomach refers to the left shoulder.

How did I know why these people have very different symptoms, very different presentations, but have the same simple issue? I was able to look at their entire health history, their diet, what has worked, what hasn't worked and put the whole picture together and figure out what is going on for each of them.

On the other side of that, a lot of people come to me because they don't have answers, there are no treatments for what's going on with them.

Arthritis is very common, so specialized medicine says well, it's just genetic, there's nothing we can do about it, here are some drugs, and let's try some therapy and see if that helps. But on the functional medicine side, we get to determine why is this happening? Is it an autoimmune issue? Is it an infection? Is it a nutritional deficiency? Heavy metals, thyroid, IBS, there's so many different reasons that someone might have an overall symptom case like arthritis that we have to figure out why, why is that person struggling with these symptoms?

I think it is important at this point in our story to address that fact that you can use the best of both worlds with traditional medicine and natural solutions. You don't have to choose one over the other and it is important to find a physician who listens to you and is willing to help you find the best plan for your body.

Putting the pieces together begins with what we have covered to this point:
Stop - Stop chasing supplements and plans
Test - Utilize testing to see what is actually going on with your body
Assess - Take a global look at your symptoms

Part of the functional assessment is a symptom overview. This is a great way to observe all of your symptoms and each category is related to a body system. I utilize this survey and others to evaluate which area of the body needs the most support since many symptoms overlap many systems. Go back to the last chapter and take the quiz!

You might be struggling with a variety of vague symptoms such as itchy skin, fatigue, headaches, joint pain, and irritable bowel syndrome. These symptoms will give you many different diagnoses depending on the doctor you see for treatment. One person might say adrenal fatigue, another might test for arthritis, one might send you for therapy, and another would say to exercise more. Which one is right?

The next steps after you assess your symptoms and body systems are:
Make a plan - work closely with a functional medicine physician and your health team
Practice - Work your plan and be willing to try different options to see what fits your body best

The best rule is to be patient, for every year you have been struggling with a specific health issue you can expect one month to recover. This isn't always true, but you can expect that as you solve one problem or symptom a new ones appear for you to heal. You can work on each layer one at a time and be joyful when a new issue shows up because you are continuing to heal on deeper levels.

Chapter 4: The Real You

Well, what did you expect?

No really, what do you expect? Do you think you will heal your body? Do you think you will be consistent this time? Do you think that there is a magic answer out there for you?

The questions of what's wrong with me, why can't I feel better, why is nothing working are just the superficial questions we ask when deep down we aren't ready to heal or face the truth of our situation.

This chapter is dedicated to you, your soul, your mind, your ego, your fears, and your dreams. Why are you not reaching your goals, what holds you back, and why you can't be consistent.

A few years ago I was working with a difficult client who we just couldn't find answers for her struggles. Every time we got close a different system shut down, or she lost composure during her period, or a family drama came up.

Seriously, even traditional and functional test came back normal. I sat down with my journal and I asked "why are these women so unhappy and stuck in the same cycles? This has to be the reason I can't reach through to her or find the right plan!"

Many women I work with struggle deeply with perfectionism, they are obsessed with their weight and size, they are terrified of their very existence.

Deep down they don't believe they are worthy or deserving of healing.

This shame, guilt, and fear keeps their body in a cycle of pain and inflammation, quite literally with neurotransmitters, cortisol, and immune shut down.

Women make up 75% of those diagnosed with autoimmune conditions, costing $100 billion annually for health care costs and it takes over 4 years to be diagnosed! Women are emotionally stressing and hating themselves to death through autoimmune diseases. They are thinking thoughts of such deep self hate and loathing to the point their body begins to attack itself.

Most women who go through my programs are able to reach a level where they are 75% better but never make it past this point. They continue to struggle with the same issues even though I know in my heart that they could experience full health. The only thing that is holding them back is their addiction to stress, perfectionism, and self criticism. This is the most important aspect of your life to heal above all things.

No supplement, pill, or treatment exists that will cure what ails you if you truly believe that you do not deserve to live your best life for yourself. If traveling for work is literally causing you physical pain, IBS, and migraines, then it is time to stop, assess, and find a different way. You can not supplement your way out of a stressful life to get to feeling good.

Women are unhappy, overwhelmed, overstressed, and constantly comparing their lives to others. We struggle with parenting and knowing what is right and wrong for our children. Every step feels like a mistake waiting to happen, a regret waiting to be fulfilled, a disaster that will have to be explained.

We don't have time to pause, relax, exist, or practice self care because we are so obsessed with stress, perfection, keeping the house clean, making sure everyone else is happy, and keeping our superficial life looking amazing.

On the inside women are dying a slow death. They don't know who they are as a person, a woman, mom, wife, sister, daughter, lover, or friend. Each role has different expectations and rules, and ones that we can't keep up with. And this is showing up as chronic illness and pain.

This is where we ignore our own health. The subtle screams for help from your body that go ignored until you're dragging yourself off the floor. Everyone and everything is more important and if you stop for one second you know that the whole world will end, everyone will judge you and hate you, and my god why can't you just lose weight like a normal person?

It doesn't help that you're chasing the wrong goals.

You want to lose weight, you won't be happy until you hit that perfect size or fit in that dress again. You can't be happy and definitely can't have sex again until you are 'perfect'. But that day never comes where you are the weight that is good enough for you or you never lose weight or worse, you start to gain weight. You keep putting more and more pressure on your body, your meals, your workouts, your family so you can reach these goals but you're unhappy, you're stressed, and no one wants to be around you. I have worked with women who made a pact with their husband they would not have sex again until they both reached their goal weight.

It is truly exhausting and crushing to feel ashamed about your weight 24/7 and carrying not only the weight but also the emotional pain. This is a pain that you can release and experience life through play, joy, and fun.

Go back to step one and stop. Take the time to journal:
In my work with women, I have come to see that the journey of health is more about becoming acceptable than it is about true health. It is better to be a size 4 than to live without migraines.

I can't answer this question for you but I can offer you a starting point. Take this time to journal and ask yourself these questions. Think about the end goal and how you want to feel when you have reached your destination. Then what is underneath these goals? Keep asking yourself why and be curious about your hopes, fears, dreams, and needs.

- Why are you chasing these goals, this number on the scale, this vision of beauty?
- What are you trying to prove?
- Who are you trying to make happy?
- What are the rules that you have created around your health, body, shape?

Is your true, deep down, super scary to admit end goal to:
-Be good enough? Good enough for who? Who made these rules?
-Grab attention?
-Prove you are worthy of love?
-Avoid rejection, isolation, or abandonment?

All these answers that you discover within yourself will give you the answers to why you aren't able to find healing or reach your goals.

Every person struggles with being consistent with their diet, food choices, going to the gym, remembering to drink water, everyone is guilty of falling off their plan at some point.

Let's just admit right now that inconsistency does not mean you are a bad person, that you are unreliable or untrustworthy, or that you shouldn't keep trying. There is nothing wrong with you and you need to start observing your patterns to discover why you choose your actions.

The number one theme I see with my clients is punishment.

Women starve themselves as punishment for their weight and size.
Some overeat as punishment for the same feelings. Many women use exercise as a punishment to their body.

Some avoid exercise because there is too much guilt for never moving in the first place.
Other women work themselves into a frenzy because they don't want to be called lazy.
Some women are shamed by friends and family for not eating sweets and candy!
Mother's use their children as an excuse to eat junk because their schedules are crazy.

This underlying theme of punishment, self loathing, and shame creates the opportunity for you to subconsciously sabotage all of your hard work.

Take some time to journal:
- Are you punishing yourself or your body? How? Why?
- How do you feel after your punish yourself with food, exercise, etc?
- How would you feel if you could stop punishing yourself?
- What would that day look like? How would you act or treat yourself?
- What is one step that you can take today to stop the cycle?

Chapter 5: Everyone Else

The worst part about doing the internal work on your mindset and beliefs is that you have to go back out into the world and exist within your relationships.

Now is the time to address the external relationships and how they are affecting your health, your ability to heal, and move forward with your life.

In this chapter we will examine the relationships throughout your life that have created stories, beliefs, and stress around how you experience your body and health. Exploring these relationships will help you uncover the root of your answers to the journaling questions in chapter 4.

When Tracy started working with me she was overweight by 100 pounds, fatigued, and had migrating pains throughout her body. As she progressed through her program it became clear during her consults that she was deeply unhappy and wasn't able to stick to any portion of her plan.

Her husband said she just needed to eat less and monitored her food. Her mom said it was all in her head, she was fine at the last family event, why can't she just get it together? Her trainer said she could eat whatever she wanted as long as it fit her macros, even if that meant pizza and fruit snacks. Her doctor said that her blood work looked great and refused to run different tests because he was sure nothing was wrong, but prescribed her thyroid medication and cholesterol drugs just in case. Even when she did stick to the plan her friends encouraged her to cheat to feel good about herself and have fun.

She had no sex drive and she was just fine with that because she fell asleep on the couch and avoided connection with her husband at all costs. She did live for her children to make sure they were at the right sport on the right day, and separated herself from the world to focus on them and her work.

She was shutting down all areas of her life while punishing herself over her weight. She actually told me "As long as I see the weight go down I'll be happy with the program" and completely ignored all of the true health issues that she was struggling to survive. You could see the light going out in her soul while she obsessed with stress, weight, perfection, and presenting a false persona to the world.

She only started to heal once she addressed the personal beliefs she had about her worth and deserving health and life, and made the connections to how she was raised with food and started to shed the layers of family stories and pain. Tracy's main connection to the secret of overcoming her health was addressing the stories she learned from her mother through counseling and journaling.

She realized that she had internalized her mom's struggle with weight and an unhappy marriage. She frantically cleaned and kept every one busy but never stopped to care for herself. The first step Tracy took was to take time off of work and focus on herself. She read books, started float sessions, and asked for help to get her kids to their sports games. Only then was she able to focus on food, supplements, and sleep.

Does Tracy's story sound familiar to you?

Healing the woman within is about discovering and then expressing your true self. Your soul, your passions, your lust for life and allowing your power to shine through. Honestly, everyone finds that concept terrifying and if you don't, then you haven't discovered your true self yet.

Healing The Mother Wound

Dr. Oscar Serrallach's work initiated the conversation about his term, the mother wound, as a way to describe how stories, beliefs, and pain are passed down through generations of women. He discusses the concept of how women are trapped in comparison of each other, feelings of being not good enough, and how mothers suppress their daughter's growth either from fear or jealousy.

Young girls are exposed to criticism at a young age through being forced to partake in their mother's struggles and journey. They are dragged to weight loss meetings, they are forced to drink protein shakes instead of eating dinner, they are weighed every day and ridiculed for their body type. As these young girls reach puberty the changes in their body are pointed out "look at your thighs!" and they are compared to other young girls.

Women are trapped in a struggle of wanting to please their mother's while at the same time find their own voice, life, and body. Bethany Webster gives us Stereotypes that perpetuate the Mother Wound:

- "Look at everything your mother did for you!" (from other people)
- "My mother sacrificed so much for me. I would be so selfish to do what she could not do. I don't want to make her feel bad."

- "I owe loyalty to my mother no matter what. If I upset her, she will think I don't value her."

I ask my patients these questions when we uncover their mother wound that is preventing their healing and I would encourage you to journal on these questions as well:
- Do you enjoy being a mom?
- Did your mom enjoy being a mom?
- How did your mom impact your view of your body and health?
- What areas did your mom struggle with in her own life?
- What does your version of an enjoyable motherhood look like?
- What values would you like to pass on to your children?

Young mothers are often stressed and unable to care for their own health while juggling everything that has to be done. They are obsessed with perfection, stress, chores, and order and they individually have to discover where the need to feel high levels of stress came from.

Many women find that they neglect their family to complete chores that will never be done. Taking the kids to the park or the zoo is a soul-sucking chore. Everything is exhausting but they have to keep pushing beyond their body's limits. There is so much shame with being imperfect and the social media comparison stress is real.

I will say it again: Most women who go through my programs are able to reach a level where they are 75% better but never make it past this point. They continue to struggle with the same issues even though I know in my heart that they could experience full health. The only thing that is holding them back is their addiction to stress, perfectionism, and self-criticism. This is the most important aspect of your life to heal above all things.

Healing Ancestral Trauma

While everyone is running to get the latest gene test done to see what they can blame for their health issues, no one has called grandma and asked her about her health. Your grandmother's experiences and exposures are much more important because that is what has affected your genes to express or not express health.

Your genetic health began with your grandmother while she was pregnant with your mother. When females are born their ovaries most of the eggs that they will carry over a lifetime. This means that you were an egg in your mother's ovary while your grandmother was pregnant with her.

The big picture means that anything your grandmother experienced during her pregnancy with your mother directly affected you as an egg. Exposures to toxins, drugs, alcohol, chemicals, and stress, emotions, abuse, or infections could directly affect your mother and you as an egg. Take some time to review your family medical history to find the hidden clues to your own health.

Ancestral healing also addresses the energetic, emotional, and cultural patterns that we inherit from our family. Women's intuition and empathic abilities allow us to innately tap into these stories and take them on as our own. We feel our mother's and grandmother's struggles and often rush to heal them while not having the emotional capability to process these emotions ourselves so they become stuck in our own body.

We become surrogates for our family stories keeping the drama alive because we don't know anything else. Women have miscarriages because the mother or other family members were unable to become pregnant easily or they didn't want to become mothers, so they subconsciously resonate with this story of being unable to fulfill a pregnancy. Work becomes all encompassing because we are taught that we must work hard and sacrifice because our families sacrificed for us. Nothing is easy and if life is easy for you then you are a cheater and a liar. These are strong and real stories that impact your health, your cells, your emotions, and how you feel your life must be lived.

Examining these stories and beliefs will help you navigate your own health struggles and release them. This will also help you avoid passing these harmful beliefs to your own children.

To heal this aspect of your life journal on where you may be surrogating for your family members and ask yourself what you need to say to them to be released from these stories.

Another topic of ancestral healing that is a big focus right now is genetics. You are not ruled by your genetics in all aspects. You do have the ability to turn on and off genes by taking excellent care of your health. The environment you are exposed to on a daily basis has more of a determining factor in how your body expresses health. Your choices with foods, sleep, stress, home and work environment, water, and practically every aspect of your life can directly impact your genes and how your body feels.

Spouse And Romantic Relationships
Your sex drive is low and you don't care. Your husband cares but at this point, he knows to just stay away. You feel rejected but also okay with that because you don't want sex anyways. You think about your body, weight, cellulite, stretch marks, and wonder if you will ever feel sexy again.

Or your sex drive is high but you have this nagging feeling that something is off and you can't explain it. I often hear "if it lasts longer than ten minutes I don't want it".

Your husband doesn't understand why you are always so stressed and can never relax. You tell him it's because women's brains are more efficient and you have 1,000 thoughts for one of his and you just can't stop thinking and worrying. He does his best to support you even though his suggestions work great for him and he lost weight but everything he tells you to do causes you to gain weight and you are both frustrated with each other.

A few years ago I was very excited about the newest research on intermittent fasting. I couldn't wait to incorporate it into our daily routine and watch those pounds melt away! My husband immediately felt great and lost 10 pounds. I immediately was starving, hangry, and gained 15 pounds. How could this be possible? I did everything right! Except when reading the research and seeing that they only have ever tested fasting on men and postmenopausal women. Those two body types do not apply to me!

I had to go the opposite direction and eat every two hours based on my body's needs at that time, which was frustrating for my husband because our eating schedules didn't overlap.

It took a few months but we finally managed to get our whole house on a supportive and individual eating plan.

The first thing we have to address is that your spouse, assuming he is a male, has a completely different physiology and what works for him will not work for you. It actually doesn't matter what gender your spouse is, you still have a different physiology! You have to forge your own path and be cheerleaders and not judges for each other.

I ask my patients about their libido because it tells me how their hormones and brain are functioning. It's always a great day when I hear someone's libido is back and everyone is happy!

Many times the root cause of low libido or disinterest in sex is about pituitary and adrenal fatigue which disrupts all of the hormones in a woman's body. The natural cycles and flow of hormones are disrupted, ovulation is painful or isn't occurring, periods are painful and heavy. When we address this root cause and allow the brain to start coordinating hormones in a healthy rhythm the desire for connection returns.

But when we talk about healing the woman within we find that there is an aspect of our self-expression that is missing. Feminine sexuality is layered with shame, guilt, pain, trauma, and fear.

I have had many conversations about the 50 Shades phenomena and how women are finding aspects of their sexuality and desires that they never thought possible but are still afraid to openly express their desires. Many women don't know what they desire until they read it in a book or online. A helpful tool is the sexual limits list that you can easily find on the internet. Print a copy and bring it to your spouse and see what you might both like to experience together.

Most women don't fully discover and express their sexuality until they learn that the female body can have 16 different TYPES of orgasms and once you being to explore these different types, what your body enjoys and prefers, and how to allow them to happen, sex is a completely different experience.

My favorite technique for women to connect to their body is daily breast massage. The Taoist deer massage is an excellent tool to increase lymph flow to drain the breasts and heart, but it also allows you to take the time every day to connect to your body, awaken your sexuality, and feel good about yourself. You can use fractionated coconut oil with clary sage or lavender for the massage or even use rose lotion.

Start by sitting with your heel resting against your clitoris. If you can't reach your heel up you can use a tennis ball. This will help increase the energy flow within your body. In circular motions massage the whole breast in one motion. You will go in both directions, clockwise and counter-clockwise. In each direction do at least 36 rotations.

Inner thigh massage either daily or as foreplay with favorite blend because of pressure points will also help lymph and blood flow. You can do this yourself or have your partner help you.

If you aren't feeling comfortable in your own skin or are not feeling confident in your body, try diffusing cinnamon oil while you are getting dressed, taking a bath, or getting ready for your night. Cinnamon is a 'hot' or caustic oil and MUST be diluted before using topically as a massage lotion.

To focus on healing yourself through this significant relationship journal on these topics:
- What was your parent's relationship like and how does that affect your beliefs and stories around marriage or relationships?
- How does your spouse support you and where do you need more support or a change in understanding?
- What works for your spouse but isn't working for you?

- How did you learn about sex and how did that affect you as a child and young adult?
- What did you learn about yourself from past relationships and how is that affecting your current relationship?
- What is your current sex life like? What do you enjoy about it and what would you like to change?
- If you were completely confident and free what would your deepest desires look like? How would you express yourself?
- If you could tell your spouse one thing about your inner sexual being what would that be? How do you think they will react?

Family Relationships

Your extended family can certainly disrupt your ability to focus on yourself and healing. Snide comments about your weight, dress, and parenting skills usually come out during family events and you feel that you have to hide or stay quiet to just get along until you get home.

When my son was 9 months old a family member told me "You know, your husband never wanted to marry someone who got pregnant and fat". That comment destroyed me for years and though it wasn't true by anyone's sad imagination, I allowed that comment to creep into my food choices, alcohol consumption and caused much unnecessary stress in my marriage.

My husband fought it with all he could but the toxicity ate me alive. On the day I was told this, I weighed 118 pounds and was wearing a size 2 jeans, thank you breastfeeding! I had lost my pregnancy weight and another 18 pounds but I still felt unworthy of love, embarrassed to be around my family and my husband, and ashamed of how I couldn't let the statement go.

We are taught to be nice, to not lash out, to smile and just say 'oh that's just the way it is'. Until we get home and can scream behind closed doors, lash out at those closest to us, or bury it deep inside until we are sick.

The only way to create change in your family dynamic is to step into your personal power. Look back at your previous journaling about why you are working to heal yourself and see how it applies to your family as well.

Are you trying to prove you are worthy? Are you trying to prove you fit in? Do you join in on the negative talk, gossip, and anger to be accepted by your family?

You have the choice to stop suppressing yourself by becoming numb, invisible, checked-out and to start acknowledging your emotions and needs. This is the most difficult section because sometimes this means limiting time with family or walking away completely.

You can have the crucial conversations with the ones you love that may unknowingly be hurting you with their negativity or own pain.

When you are ready to acknowledge and take action on this step take some time to journal on your family. How do you feel when you are with them and after you return home? Are you a different person when you are with them and how? How are their words and actions affecting you, emotionally, physically, and in your other relationships? What would you like to be different? Where are you willing to take personal responsibility for being a part of their negative cycles and contributing to their pain as well?

Children

This section was originally going to be about how women sacrifice too much for their children and immediate family to create a false sense of being good enough and perfect enough. They sabotage their own personal health because they do everything for their children and can't ever be caught doing something for their own gain. My patient's tell me "oh I couldn't eat today because I had to drop the kids off at school, and go shopping, and then clean, and then it was time to pick up the kids again" and it's now 4pm and they refused to eat all day. Then they can't understand why they have no energy and can't get off the couch to actually enjoy being with their family.

You love your children and you would do anything for them. Please don't ever stop because there is nothing wrong with this. Making excuses to not take care of yourself is where the problem lives. Not eating, exercising, or having friends isn't worth the sacrifice because your children will see and learn these patterns. Learn to meal plan, keep snacks in the car, have your children be involved in meal planning, prep at night for your mornings and layout breakfast, clothes, and backpacks.

There is the infinite nature of housework that is soul crushing for women. You are the only one who picks up the discarded and stinky socks that are stuck under the couch. You are the only one who replaces the toilet paper roll and actually throws the old one in the trash. You carry the lists of what the home needs to function. You plan meals that no one eats. There are always dishes, laundry, and dirty underwear. You can't wait to be home but then you can't relax at home because there is guilt, shame, and fatigue layered in with the dirt.

Just for today remember that everything will always be dirty and waiting for you so just go take a bath and read a book.

Journal and ask yourself where are you sabotaging or sacrificing your health for your family? Why do you think you are allowing yourself to do this? What do you need to address in order to stop making excuses and create balance in your life? What would your family dynamic look like if you put yourself first so you can talk care of everyone else with energy?

I promise the world won't fall apart if you put yourself first. For example, if you eat breakfast WITH your children. At the end of the day, putting yourself first, or at least as the same priority as everyone else, allows your children to develop independence and learn that taking care of themselves is a priority (not that they didn't already know that) and in a healthy way.

The greatest gift to hand down to your children is the ability to trust their intuition, have a strong sense of self, and be able to act on it. Our daughters (and sons) grow up listening to how their mother talk about and treat her body and as an adult reflect those emotions and actions. When you speak about your body ask yourself is that how you want your child speaking about their body?

Our daughters are also learning from social media and friends about how to talk about their body to fit in. I was listening to my daughter with her friends and she said "ugh my thighs are so fat". I made what would probably be considered a major parenting mistake but I leapt into the room screaming "WHAT?!?! Why did you say that and where did you ever hear those words??" We talked for a little while and I completely embarrassed her with her friends but for a 10 year old girl who is a perfect and healthy size, has long and lean runners legs, to say she is fat just terrified me. We have talked about what she said and how she views her body, and she talked about how the girls in her school complain about their legs or stomachs and why.

If you have children it is important to talk to them about their own perceptions of their body for the emotional health of loving and treating their body right and it is important to recognize that they might not be saying these things in front of you so we as the mothers need to have these conversations constantly. I tell my daughter that we will have many conversations about these topics.

Giving your children the personal power to trust their body allows them to bring their concerns to you so you can best guide them. You can ask them questions like:
- What feels right or best to you?
- How does that feel in your body?

- How does that make your heart or belly feel?
- What decision would feel happy?

Use words that they are familiar and comfortable with and you will find that they begin to make healthier choices and their confidence will grow.

Community and Friends

Friendships can be some of the most toxic relationships you will ever experience and as you continue on this journey of healing you will find that as you grow, you grow away from friends and even family. You will also grow closer to those who truly love and support you, and are excited about your growth.

Toxic relationships also looks like every person who is wasting time away at the local coffee shop talking about how sick they are, the latest medications, and toenail fungus. My husband can't go with me anymore because he can't focus with all the ridiculous drama he hears around him. Your friends can be like your spouse, they have the best intentions and desperately want to help you but their advice is junk and is only working for them. Coaches, mentors, and professionals can be toxic to you as well when their values are not aligned with your own

"My friends are eating (name a diet: paleo, AIP, IF, keto) and they all lost twenty pounds!"
"My friends don't understand why you are having me eat like this"
"My nutritionist said to eat whatever I want. I can have pizza and gummy bears as long as it fits my macros"
"My coach wants me to be 12% body fat."

Feel like running away after reading these real statements from my patients? Good, because that is exactly what you should do.

As you find and follow your intuition you realize that the conversations you used to enjoy and connect through are now draining and exhausting. You don't want to talk about the news, the latest drama at the school, or hear how your friends are struggling in their marriage but not doing anything about it. You can't stand the gossip and you start to wonder if something is wrong with you! Who are you now? And who are you to think you are better than your closest friends?

Nothing is wrong with you except that you are healing and your soul is looking to the future, and a happy and healthy future. You are releasing the toxic relationships that you have with yourself, your body, your food, your family, and your friends. You are creating a whole new you! This is incredibly isolating but I promise you are not alone.

You have permission to heal, live, and express yourself. You are allowed to examine all of your relationships, including your relationship with your self and soul, and begin to dismantle the destructive behaviors, mentality, and energy. You have the right to create and uphold boundaries with others and even protect yourself when someone says something harmful or hateful.

Journaling questions and prompts:
Where do you need to have stronger boundaries and with whom?
How are your friends affecting your emotions and energy?
Who do you love spending time with, who is the person that is uplifting to you?
Are limitations placed on you because you have to comply with others in order to receive love?
If you put up healthy boundaries do you fear losing love and acceptance?

Chapter 6: Your Spirit

Healing your spirit, your soul, and the woman within feels heavy, overwhelming, and intense at first. This journey is not easy or simple, but finding yourself on the other side and creating your best life on your terms is the greatest gift you could give yourself.

This chapter is for you if you say "I don't feel good, but I'm not really that bad, I don't know, I just feel off". The point in your life where you can't find anything wrong or bad but you also can't figure out how to feel great.

My functional physician voice will say to look at both physical and spiritual aspects. Physically we look at the immune system, your barrier systems like the brain and gut, and how is your body recovering after stress. If your blood-brain barrier is compromised then you might struggle with brain fog, short term memory loss, fatigue, anxiety, and sensitivity to chemicals and foods. We can easily test and address this issue. Remember, before you jump to heal emotionally remember that you need to test and address the physical causes as well.

You are a powerful spiritual being and true health is an expression of who you truly are on a soul level and your connection to a higher source and power. This can mean specifically your religion and connection to God or can be as simple as your spiritual connection to yourself, nature, and the universe.

Women are missing a sense of purpose in their lives and are asking is this all life has to offer? They focus every second on their children and are lost and alone when their children are grown. They have no sense of self and don't' know how to exist without putting others first.

The journey of healing your spirit is a deep one that requires strength and a mature intuition. To initiate this connection it is important that you begin to clear space mentally, emotionally, and physically.

Slow down today
You have time
Time to do everything you need
Time to enjoy the day
Time to breathe and live in your body

Just for this moment
Feel into your body
Drop your awareness into your heart

And the space in front of your heart
Take 10 deep breaths
What is your body telling you today
What does your body need

There is no rush.

Connecting physical, emotional, and spiritual pain

In alternative medicine (traditional Chinese medicine, Ayurvedic, Native traditions) each body system is connected to an energy path, as in acupuncture meridians or chakras. Each path is related to an element, a physical symptom, an emotion, food, and color.

For this segment we will focus on the acupuncture system for you to understand and connect your symptoms to emotions and find a root of healing. You can also use the chakra system to connect your emotions to your physical symptoms.

The lungs control our breathing and energy, and are responsible for helping energy flow through the body. When we are feeling disappointment, grief, loss, shame, or sadness the lungs will manifest physically with issues of the chest, lung, throat, and even the sinuses. Long term grief that is not addressed consciously can impact the protective layer of the lungs.

The bladder is connected to a lack of energy, resistant to change, and having a pessimistic attitude. Bladder infections are typically met with the question of "who are you pissed off at?" and addressing the physical and emotional aspects of both.

The kidneys hold our courage and strength of will. They are affected by fear of the future, insecurity with money and relationships, and inability to make decisions. This intense fear can manifest as stones, urinary tract infections, tinnitus, hernias, and irregular menstrual cycles.

The triple warmer is a term that is the acupuncture meridian that encompasses life energy. Emotions that affect this meridian are instability and frigidity and when balanced you feel joyful and light. Physical imbalances may include the area of the body the meridian travels with the gallbladder, heart, and small intestine.

The gallbladder is strongly related to our courage and initiative. When you are feeling indecision, resentment, and fearful of decisions you may also notice physical manifestations of insomnia, neck pain, loose stools, eye dysfunction.

The liver is closely associated with creativity so feeling stuck, angry, resentment, and jealousy are emotions to check in with physically. Issues such as blurry vision is often a result of liver congestion as well as waking at 3am and not being able to fall back asleep.

The large intestine is focused on movement, like the lungs, and is also affected by grief, sadness, and worry. Physical weakness may also be a sign of large intestine dysfunction, along with low self esteem or self worth, congested lungs, and of course any digestive dysfunctions.

The heart is the queen of emotions and can be most affected by the emotions of sadness, depression, fear, loss of love, jealousy, and not following your soul purpose. Physically you will feel chest congestion, difficulty breathing, memory issues, and also throat issues.

The pericardium is the membrane that surrounds the heart and is a meridian that is the 'bodyguard'. It is sensitive to emotions like the heart, specifically depression or avoidance. Many people who have these emotions will also struggle with emotional outbursts, feeling like they are on a rollercoaster, or feel every emotion as the body tries to process through the organs.

The small intestines digest and absorb our food and emotionally the related to our ability to create and act on new ideas. Unclear or incomplete thoughts, restlessness, and the inability to share or express emotions suggests the small intestine may be affected. Physically, you may experience excessive sweating, pain in your abdomen, and bloating.

The spleen produces red blood cells and is part of our immune system. From an energetic perspective it is related to self esteem and when imbalanced can be felt as worry, excessive eating and drinking, opinionated, and stubborn. Physical manifestations include digestive and stomach pain and immune compromise.

The stomach is the focus for worry, suspicion, and concerns. The butterflies we feel may be related to our intuition and causes us experience acid reflux, distension, sore throat, or bleeding gums.

This is a list of the acupuncture meridians and their related emotions and physical manifestations. This is a list to help guide you and when you are feeling a specific emotion, to look to the organ it is related to and as well as physical pain.

If you are struggling with bloating and indigestion, look to your stomach and small intestine. Are you suppressing your creativity and not allowing yourself to follow the flow of your life? If you struggle with constant allergies or coughing, where in your life are you experiencing grief or loss?

The emotional work is supported best with physical work. You can't expect to only manage your emotional state and your body will heal. Always provide the support your body needs through nutrition, movement, supplementation and always uncover any hidden causes through testing. Never assume your emotions are the sole cause of your pain but do not discount them as a factor in your healing.

Reclaiming the pieces of your soul

Soul fragmentation occurs when there is trauma, pain, or repression of spirit. Our body continues to move forward but a part of us is missing, lost, stuck in the past or in a specific event, and we feel incomplete. This incomplete feeling causes a pressure to search outside of ourselves to become whole. We dive into abusive relationships with the promise of pleasure and love, we turn to alcohol and drugs to feel good, we isolate ourselves afraid of interacting with others to avoid pain.

Your life is numb, your experiences sterile, your relationships are cold.

Intuitive healing comes from within yourself and that is where you will find the answers. As I was writing this section and thinking about my own personal soul, I took some time off to go into meditation. I never knew how I could do this process without the designated shaman or ritual that the experts say you need.

But I remember that experts are there as guides and I decided to call on my spirit animal. I rarely ever do this, it's actually been a few years but I felt a very powerful call to just sit down and be still, let's see what happens. I'm still hesitant to write this because your own experience will be completely different and if you have made it this far in the book, well you're stuck with me now.

As I sat down to meditate on soul retrieval I had the vision of a stunningly white polar bear walk up on my left. I asked him to help me find any pieces of my soul or spirit that may be missing and he immediately took off. I followed close behind as he ran, then quickly turned right, then left, and left again. I kept thinking to myself "this is stupid, it's not real, why am I doing this" but I held on because the feelings were so strong.

When the bear stopped he was biting something on the ground. I pulled two black ravens out of his mouth and they sat on my shoulder. I had an overwhelming sense of peace and wholeness like I had never experienced before.

What does it all mean? Nothing and everything. Your experience is your own and if you have struggled spiritually and energetically, this is an opportunity to connect with your past self. Go back through your life and see yourself during times of struggle, stress, or traumatic events. Ask your soul to come back, to be healed, and return to you.

Which pieces of yourself have been left behind, forgotten, or harmed?
What age is that piece of soul that has escaped, where is it hiding, and what caused it to flee?

Spirituality is stillness, space, and self. When we speak with our higher self and tune into all the aspects of our soul we are able to become whole.

The next chapter will help you connect with your intuition but it is important to first realize that you have to first connect to yourself and your soul before you can connect on an authentic and spiritual level with your spouse, your children, and your community.

Life and Death
You are reclaiming pieces of your soul and with those fragments are memories, emotions, stories, and pain. Like a parasite or virus in your mind the old thoughts creep back in, reminding you of who you 'really are'.

But those thoughts are just that, a parasite in your mind, that lies to you and disrupts your path. They exist because they are your default settings. It is a default program to return to depression and anxiety when life starts going well. It is a default program that is comfortable, familiar, safe to live in while you forget your strength and power.

Too much power or control can feel overwhelming and scary. We see women who are powerful and the judgments that come along with that power. She shouldn't be so overtly sexual! Who is watching her kids? I can't believe she gained so much weight. Does this mean if I'm powerful and fully expressed I will be fat, divorced, and alone? No thank you!

When you call your soul back and heal the patterns within your life and your relationships you in control of what lives and what dies. You have the power to transform, restore, create, and manifest. You now have the knowledge of self alongside the power to express yourself. You get to decide who you want to be from now on, how you want to live your life, and how you want to be treated. That is an abundance of power ready for you to claim.

Your whole health and being depend on your ability to kill the parasites that cloud your body and mind with drama and pain. These parasites aren't real but are programmed to keep you safe and small.

Life and death as a topic here is about the ability to allow life in, be present, create experiences, and find joy. Death is about accepting that aspects of our lives are not meant to live forever, grieving for the loss, being grateful for the opportunity, and creating new life. Friendships, spouses, relationships, careers, businesses, homes, all pass through the cycle. Our children grow up and we grieve for the loss of the beloved stages while celebrating their growth.

Death occurs in the parts and parasites that are harmful within us. Allowing the voice of fear, uncertainty, doubt, and hate to die will allow you to plant the seeds for love, compassion, acceptance, and help you return to the life you were designed to live.

As we accept that life goes through the cycles of creation, life, death, and renewal we can focus on the balance of our energies. Women are taught to push, hustle, work, and rush. We follow the masculine energy of the world and push ourselves to exhaustion while feeling guilty for taking time to rest and heal. We sleep in and immediately regret it because of the time lost. We take time to exercise but feel bad for putting our kids in the play center.

When I left chiropractic to focus on my essential oil business I was finally given the space to sleep in and I enjoyed every second of it. I still do today. When I went to visit the networking group I was involved with as a chiropractor and obviously complaining about how early it was in the morning, a man in my networking group told me I would never be successful if I didn't start getting up early. If I didn't make the calls or execute the sales by 9am I was a failure to him. Thankfully he was incredibly wrong and I am here to tell you today that you do not have to live and judge yourself by others standards.

Women live in an amazing flow of push and pull, work and rest, hustle and vacation. The male mentors in chiropractic harshly judge by numbers, income, output, goals. The female mentors I work with focus on the flow of creativity and passion, focusing on your individual values, and enjoying your business.

We can accomplish so much more when we follow our feminine intuition of when to rest, heal, move slowly, connect to those around us and when to hustle, work hard, stay up all night blogging or coaching clients. It's all up to you and as soon as you let the 'rules' go, let the numbers go, the flow will come to you and you will feel balance.

Journal on these questions:
- Are you ready to step into your full power?
- What would your body look like if you were in control?
- How would you behave if you were 100% expressed?
- If 100% is too much how about 50% expressed?
- What do you want to kill most in your programming right now?
- How did this programming serve you and keep you safe?
- Tune in to your body and ask what is the best way to bring that program to an end?
- Where you feel imbalanced in your energy? Are you pushing or working too hard?
- What are the rules you feel you have to follow in order to be successful?

Chapter 7: Your Intuition

Tuning into your own intuition is as simple as you allow it to be.

Start with slowing down physically, emotionally, and mentally. Calm your thoughts and your breathing. Your body holds your intuition and to feel that calling you must be empty of expectations. As you are sitting or laying down, bring your awareness into your body. We spend most of our time living in our heads, emotionally in the past or the future. This requires you to live in the present and feel into your body. Feel your feet on the floor, the angle of your knees, the pressure in your hips and pelvis. Feel the muscles of your spine and core as you breathe. Feel the weight in your arms and hands. What does living in your body feel like?

Your intuition may live in different areas of your body. When you ask a question of yourself and you are looking for an answer don't look in your brain or your head. Your answers may come from your third eye/forehead, heart, hands, gut, feet, ovaries, vagina, or aura. Feel into each of these areas as you still your body and mind to see which one carries your strongest feelings.

Your intuition responses may look completely different than you expect. You may expect a gut reaction, a feeling or sensation in your body, others will hear a voice giving them answers, some will smell or taste, others will have a knowing.

The best place to start when tuning into your body and soul is to look for the feeling of contraction of energy, tightening or constricting in your body, or a sinking feeling as the answer of no. The feeling of rising or expanding energy is the answer of yes. You may hear or feel the answer of yes or no as well but always follow the feeling within your body as that is your true answer.

As you continue to follow the contraction or expansion energy as your soul's guidance and direction you will find that you are always on the right path though it might not consciously make sense to you at the time.

Asking questions is the foundation of a mature intuition. Questioning allows you to evaluate, decide, protect, and create. The inquisitive nature of women has always been labeled as snooping, nosey, annoying and as we have been taught to suppress our natural instincts to explore and feel into situations we have killed off our innate ability to protect ourselves.

As young children we are taught to be still, be pretty, and don't talk about the difficult or bad things we see. Everyone is happy, everything is great. We muffle our screams to escape pain and abuse to keep others around us satisfied that all is well. Instead of living our life with strength, confidence, and knowledge we have cut ourselves off from our power, our gifts, and created a shallow, false, and painful life.

If you find stillness a difficult concept to feel into your body and soul then get up and try something different. There are no rules or judgments in the way you connect to yourself! Prayer, meditation, dancing, drumming, singing, painting, writing, lovemaking, anything that connects you (while sober) to an altered state will help you tune in. Emptiness in your body, mind, and heart allows the messages you need to hear and feel be experienced strongly and without doubt.

There is peace and stillness to be found in expansion, growth, movement, and restlessness of your spirit. When you find yourself disconnected or out of flow with your inner guidance use this as a sign to re-evaluate your plan for the moment. Release any judgement around the frustration in the lack of response.

We have all been there, wondering if we will ever hear the call of our soul again, wondering if we will be alone forever. But you know that isn't true, you are not lost and alone. Change your environment, connect with others, and find inspiration. Allow your mind and soul to wander and play, give yourself new experiences. When you return and are ready to connect again you will have ideas to respond to and find that expansion feeling with a new idea.

When you venture into the dark you will have no fear because your soul is your light to carry you through with truth and love. Healing your soul will heal your body as your soul's journey flows through your life like a river.

"Until you make the unconscious conscious, it will direct your life and you will call it fate."
― C.G. Jung

What happens when you do all of these things but still don't hear or feel the calling of your intuition? Check in with each body part or system and check where your body is holding trauma, shame, or pain. If your ovaries are the seat of your intuition like it is for many women, but you resist pleasure, love, acceptance, orgasm, or connection, you are cut off from the very source of your intuition. Treat your ovaries with love, massage, yoni steam, or even just talk with them and ask what they need to heal. The answer may surprise you.

When you open these doors of your body and soul, the feelings and situations you encounter may be painful and dark. Stay awake and stay alert and resist the temptation to hide from this pain. Once this door is unlocked and the truth is revealed will follow you and stay alive until it is met head-on, consciously dealt with action and intuitive force. Seek support from your trusted relations, seek supportive counseling, and allow these aspects of your life and soul to heal.

Another tool to help you integrate your intuition and follow your soul's guidance is Human Design. Human Design has been an invaluable tool for my personal and professional life. This is a concept developed around our genetics, birth date, and authentic nature. There are 4 "Types" and each Type has a specific set of instructions on how to ask for, feel into, and act on their intuition. For more information visit www.jovianarchive.com.

The last steps we will discuss in this chapter are caring for your inner world through your physical body, and connecting with nature. Grounding is a technique that is simply connecting with the ground. This allows your body to transfer electrons and reduce free radicals.
This simply means walking barefoot or sitting on the ground for an extended time. My best health is expressed when I spend spring and summer afternoons on the lawn reading while my children play outside.

When it is too cold to go play we use a grounding mat. I find it helpful to place the mat under my feet while working at my desk and also while I am sleeping.

Creating and allowing space to retreat, heal, and sleep is the biggest key in developing and feeling your intuition. On this healing path you may find that you require more sleep, naps, and downtime. You may find that you are bursting with creative energy as you peel off karmic and ancestral layers. You are free to dance through life. You may find that your dreams are becoming more vivid and meaningful or you may find that your dreams have completely stopped.

There are no right or wrong expressions of your soul work, focus on heeding what your body is asking for. Move when it is time to move, rest when it is time to rest. Keep asking yourself what you need in this moment and always listen and follow through on the answer.

Caring for your inner world requires a few steps. First is to clear out your emotional and spiritual home. Acknowledge and release anything that has been creating negative space for you.
Clearing can look like taking a bath or shower, washing your hair and face, cleaning or organizing your home. Physically clearing space will emotionally and energetically clear space, even if that means just one room that you will be resting in.

My husband knows when I am stressed because I rearrange all the furniture because it helps me re-organize my thoughts as well. I am lucky enough to have a large closet and I like to organize there and then use the space to meditate and journal. It's much easier than trying to clean the whole house first!

After you clear space it is time to sort your thoughts. Most people jump into meditation expecting to clear their mind immediately and leave frustrated after 2 minutes because their inner voice never quiets. Take some time to feed your body and mind first. You can create a ritual of clearing space physically, bringing a glass of water or tea and your journal, and write down your current thoughts, struggles, excitements, and pain. Write down the words or phrases that you hear your inner voice or judgmental voice saying to you.

As you write them down you will begin to see the patterns and the specific thoughts you can release or build upon. Writing will also help to clear your emotions and thoughts so you can take some time after in prayer or meditation without disruption. You can build upon the positive emotions and desires at this time or even quiet yourself to hear your true intuition and subconscious come through.

You can take this time to ask your body questions and wait for the answer. Keep your journal close to you so you don't forget any answers that are brought forth. There is no right or wrong in clearing your body and mind, each person has their own paths and rituals.

Chapter 8: The Unending Journey

There is no end goal, no tape at the end of the race to break through when you are healing yourself. I wish there was a way I could say "done!" for you, you're healed, you're perfect, and you are free to eat ice-cream for breakfast, lunch, and dinner. From now on, your relationships will be easy, your children will be happy, and you are complete.

I can tell you that you are never lost and alone, though you may feel that way throughout your life. Look for the lighthouse of your soul, your intuition, and continue to build that relationship.

As I was writing this book I definitely felt hypocritical. When was the last time I checked in with myself or actually acted on that physical feeling of expansion or contraction? I go through my own life and death cycles and when life is going good I often forget to check in, follow my guidance, and soon enough I'm lost in the ocean wondering how I got there.

Using my intuition may have saved my life because I was able to keep digging and find the answers to my fatigue and pain. I might have seriously done harm with the supplements I was taking and the path I was living. But when I tuned in, ignored those around me even though I was terrified to, I always had the answer in front of me.

It is safe to trust yourself and follow your own path. It will look different than the path of others, you will feel and act different, but that is the right and real path for you. Don't give up and don't stop seeking.

To living your best life,

Dr. Alison DiBarto Goggin

About The Author

Since 2005, Dr. Alison DiBarto Goggin has been studying and practicing nutrition, applied kinesiology, Reiki, and functional medicine. She graduated from Logan College of Chiropractic in 2009. She resides in Saint Louis, Missouri with her husband and two children.

She believes that every woman deserves to have the energy, passion, and health to enjoy their family and life by utilizing self-care and a wellness lifestyle. She specializes in women's health care, thyroid and hormone support, and IBS/SIBO issues and creates a customized healing program for each client.

Little Black Bag Medicine is a functional wellness practice that offers flexible telemedicine and phone or video consultations. Your consultations are completed at a convenient time for you either during lunch or after your children are in bed. Lab testing is available including blood, saliva, and hair with an extensive selection of options. Testing kits can be sent to your home making testing in the privacy of your home easy and simple. Test results are reviewed over the phone along with your personalized plan.

You can find out more about working with Dr. DiBarto-Goggin through individual consultations and programs at www.LittleBlackBagMedicine.com

Works Cited

Bissell, M.g. "Establishing Reference Intervals for Clinical Laboratory Test Results: Is There a Better Way?" *Yearbook of Pathology and Laboratory Medicine*, vol. 2011, 2011, pp. 240–241., doi:10.1016/s1077-9108(10)79506-2.

"Scientific Research: Health Benefits of Personal Grounding/Earthing." *Groundology*, www.groundology.co.uk/scientific-research.

"Why It's Crucial for Women to Heal the Mother Wound." *Womb of Light*, womboflight.com/why-its-crucial-for-women-to-heal-the-mother-wound.

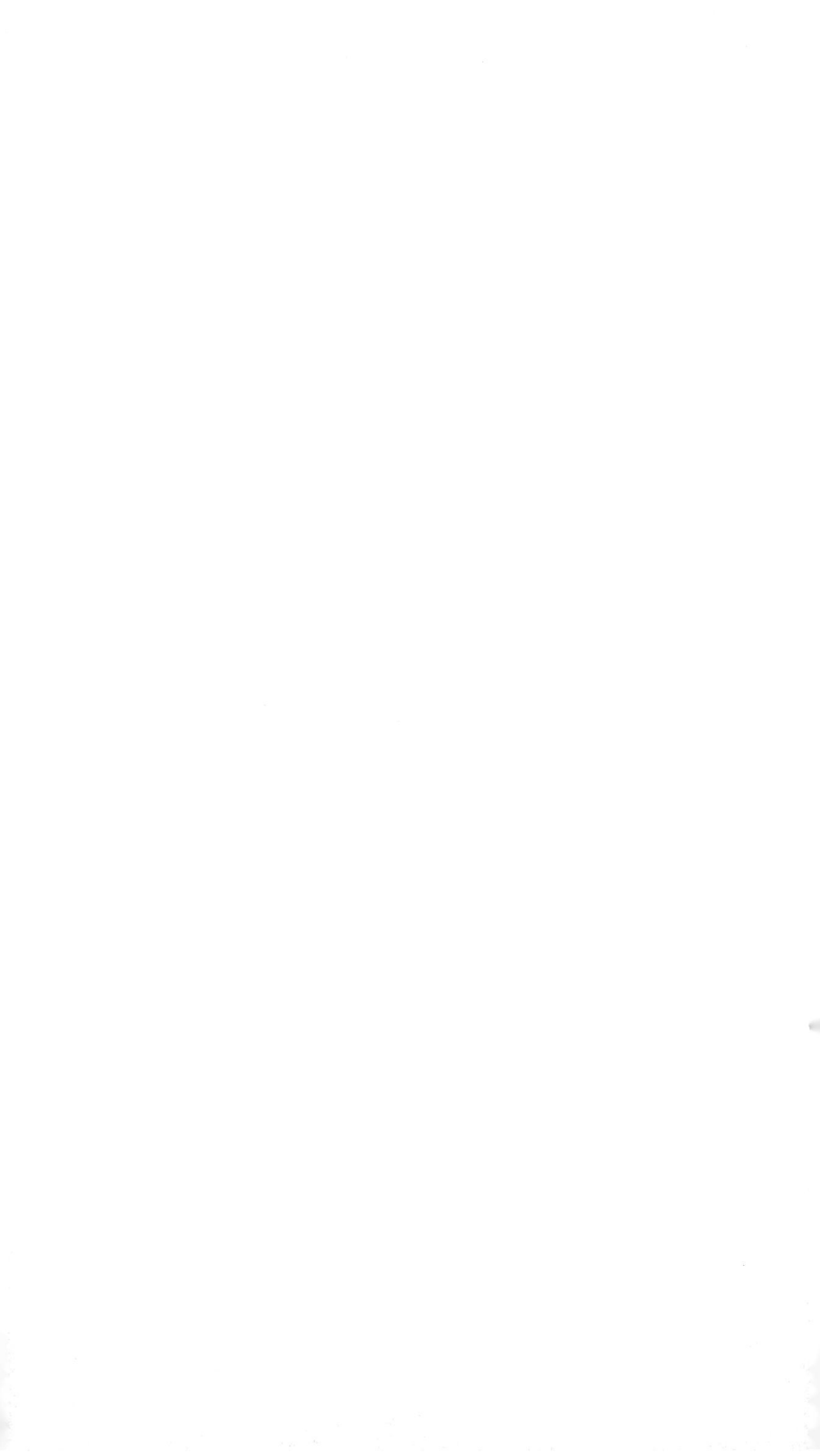

Made in the USA
Lexington, KY
13 January 2019